ACHIEVING BALANCE

Navigating the Acid Reflux Diet Lifestyle

Tim A. Nakashima

TABLE OF CONTENTS

CHAPTER 6

Everyday Acid Reflux Management

CONCLUSION

The Challenges of Living with Acid Reflux

INTRODUCTION

Hello everyone! If you're looking for relief from acid reflux, you've come to the right place. Acid reflux can be a painful and disruptive condition, but the good news is that a balanced diet can make a big difference in managing symptoms. In this book, "Achieving Balance: Navigating the Acid Reflux Diet Lifestyle," we'll explore how understanding your personal triggers, focusing on nourishing foods, and making lifestyle changes can help you achieve lasting relief from acid reflux. So, let's get started on your journey towards a healthier and more balanced life!

Acid reflux affects millions of people worldwide, causing discomfort and pain on a daily basis. The condition is caused by stomach acid flowing back into the esophagus, leading to symptoms such as heartburn, belching, and difficulty swallowing. The standard treatment for acid reflux often involves medication, but did you know that a balanced diet can also make a big impact in managing symptoms?

In this book, "Achieving Balance: Navigating the Acid Reflux Diet Lifestyle," we'll explore the connection between what you eat and how you feel. We'll start by discussing the essentials of the acid reflux diet, including the foods to focus on and the foods to avoid. You'll learn how to identify your personal triggers and how to keep a food and symptom journal. You'll also discover delicious and healthy recipes to help you feel your best, along with tips for meal planning and preparation.

In addition to dietary changes, we'll also explore the role of lifestyle factors such as stress, sleep, physical activity, and smoking in managing acid reflux. We'll provide practical tips for coping with these challenges and for working with your healthcare team. Finally, we'll discuss how to stay committed to the acid reflux diet and how to celebrate your successes along the way.

So, if you're ready to take control of your acid reflux and achieve lasting balance, let's get started. Remember, the journey towards a healthier and more balanced life starts with just one step.

CHAPTER 1

Introduction to Acid Reflux and the Importance of a Balanced Diet

Acid reflux is a widespread digestive disorder that affects millions of individuals worldwide. It occurs when the lower esophageal sphincter (LES), the valve that separates the stomach from the esophagus, relaxes at the wrong time, allowing stomach acid to flow back into the esophagus. This can result in a sensation of burning in the chest and throat, also known as heartburn. Acid reflux can also cause belching, difficulty swallowing, and a sour taste in the mouth, in addition to heartburn.

Although medication is frequently used to treat acid reflux, a healthy diet can also play an important role in managing symptoms. This chapter will examine the fundamentals of acid reflux, the significance of a balanced diet, and the objectives of the acid reflux diet.

Understanding Acid Reflux

When the LES relaxes at the wrong time, stomach acid flows back into the esophagus, causing acid reflux. This may occur following a meal, while lying down, or even while sleeping. The stomach acid irritates the esophageal lining, causing symptoms such as heartburn, belching, and difficulty swallowing.

In some instances, acid reflux can also result in complications such as esophagitis, Barrett's esophagus, and even esophageal cancer. It is essential to seek medical attention if you experience frequent or persistent acid reflux symptoms, as they may indicate more serious health issues.

Acid Reflux: The Importance of a Balanced Diet

A balanced diet is essential for acid reflux management. By modifying your diet, you can reduce the frequency and severity of symptoms. This is particularly helpful for those who experience occasional acid reflux, as lifestyle changes such as dietary modifications are frequently sufficient to provide relief.

In addition to aiding in the management of symptoms, a balanced diet can promote overall health and well-being. By consuming nourishing foods, you can provide your body with the nutrients it requires to function at its best. This can also aid in reducing inflammation and enhancing digestion, both of which can improve acid reflux management.

The Objectives of an Acid Reflux Diet

The purpose of the acid reflux diet is to alleviate symptoms and prevent acid reflux-related damage. By altering your diet, you can reduce the amount of acid your stomach produces and the number of triggers that cause acid reflux. This can reduce the frequency and severity of symptoms and improve overall health and wellness.

The acid reflux diet can reduce the risk of complications such as esophagitis, Barrett's esophagus, and esophageal cancer in addition to managing symptoms. By adhering to a nutritious and well-balanced diet, you can manage your acid reflux and enhance your quality of life.

Understanding the fundamentals of acid reflux and the significance of a well-balanced diet are the first steps in managing symptoms and achieving lasting relief. In the following chapter, we'll examine the relationship between acid reflux and individual triggers and learn how to identify your own.

CHAPTER 2

<u>Understanding Your Acid Reflux Triggers and Keeping a Food and Symptom Journal</u>

In this chapter, we will examine the relationship between acid reflux and individual triggers and learn how to identify your own. By identifying the causes of your symptoms, you can make dietary and lifestyle modifications to reduce the frequency and severity of acid reflux.

Identifying Personal Triggers

Personal triggers are the particular foods, beverages, and lifestyle factors that can cause acid reflux symptoms. These may include fatty or spicy foods, caffeine, alcohol, stress, and even stress.

Keeping a food and symptom diary is the most effective way to identify your personal triggers. You will record what you eat, when you eat it, and any symptoms that occur within two hours of eating in this journal. This can assist you in identifying patterns and correlations between your diet and your symptoms, allowing you to make informed dietary and lifestyle adjustments.

Keeping a Journal of Diet and Symptoms

To begin a food and symptom journal, you will require a notebook and a pen. If you prefer, you can also use a smartphone app or an online tool. You will record the following information in your journal:

The time and date of every meal and snack
What you consumed for food and drink
The size of each food item's serving
Symptoms occurring within two hours of a meal
It is essential to be as precise and specific as possible when keeping a food and symptom journal. The more information you have, the easier it will be to identify your personal triggers and implement targeted dietary and lifestyle modifications.

Utilizing Your Food and Symptom Record

After a few days or weeks of keeping a food and symptom journal, you can begin to search for patterns and correlations between your diet and your symptoms. For instance, you may observe that you always experience heartburn after eating spicy foods or that drinking coffee causes you to belch every time.

Once you've identified your individual acid reflux triggers, you can make dietary and lifestyle modifications to reduce the frequency and severity of acid reflux symptoms. If you find that coffee always causes you to belch, you could try switching to decaf coffee or limiting your coffee consumption to a certain time of day.

It is also important to discuss your personal acid reflux triggers and other risk factors with your healthcare team. They can offer additional support and guidance, as well as assist you in developing a personalized plan for managing your acid reflux symptoms.

Identifying personal acid reflux triggers is an essential step in reducing the frequency and severity of acid reflux symptoms. You can gain control over your acid reflux and improve your quality of life by keeping a food and symptom diary and making targeted changes to your diet and lifestyle.

In addition to keeping a food and symptom diary, there are additional methods for identifying your personal triggers. For instance, you can try an elimination diet, in which you eliminate certain foods from your diet for a period of time and then reintroduce them one by one to determine if they trigger symptoms. This can be an effective method for identifying food sensitivities and allergies that may be contributing to acid reflux.

Pay attention to physical activities that may trigger your acid reflux symptoms as a second strategy. For instance, lying down or exercising shortly after eating can cause stomach acid to reflux into the esophagus. You can try avoiding physical activity for several hours after a meal, or you can choose gentle exercise over more strenuous activities.

Another common trigger for acid reflux symptoms is stress. The relaxation of the sphincter muscle at the top of the stomach, which allows stomach acid to reflux into the esophagus, can be caused by stress. By practicing relaxation techniques such as meditation, yoga, deep breathing, and progressive muscle relaxation, stress can be reduced.

In addition to these strategies, there are lifestyle modifications that can help reduce the likelihood of acid reflux symptoms. For instance, quitting smoking and avoiding secondhand smoke, losing weight if overweight or obese, and avoiding clothing that puts pressure on the abdomen.

Remember that everyone's experience with acid reflux is different, and what works for one person may not work for another. Therefore, it is essential to keep a food and symptom diary and collaborate with your healthcare team to develop a personalized plan for acid reflux management. You

can achieve balance and reduce your symptoms
with the right combination of diet, lifestyle changes,
and medical support.

CHAPTER 3

<u>Foods to Focus On and Foods to Avoid</u>

In this chapter, we will discuss the foods to emphasize and avoid on the acid reflux diet. The purpose of the acid reflux diet is to reduce the frequency and severity of acid reflux symptoms by avoiding or limiting trigger foods and increasing the consumption of foods that are gentle on the digestive system.

Foods to Emphasise

The following foods should form the basis of a diet for acid reflux:

Whole Grains: Whole grains such as brown rice, quinoa, and whole wheat bread are high in fiber and can help reduce acid reflux symptoms by promoting regular bowel movements and decreasing stomach acid.

Chicken, fish, and tofu are lean protein sources that are low in fat and gentle on the digestive system. By reducing the amount of acid in the stomach, they can alleviate the symptoms of acid reflux.

Low-Acid Fruits: Low-acid fruits, such as bananas, melons, and berries, are gentle on the digestive system and neutralize stomach acid, thereby reducing acid reflux symptoms.

Vegetables: Because they are high in fiber and low in acid, leafy greens, broccoli, and carrots are an excellent option for people with acid reflux. By promoting regular bowel movements and neutralizing stomach acid, they can reduce symptoms.

Avoidable Dietary Ingredients

The following foods should be avoided or consumed in moderation:

Fatty and Spicy Foods: Fatty and spicy foods can increase stomach acid production, leading to acid reflux symptoms.

Tomatoes and Citrus Fruits Tomatoes and citrus fruits are rich in acid, which can irritate the digestive tract and cause acid reflux symptoms.

Caffeine: Caffeine can increase stomach acid production, leading to acid reflux symptoms.

Alcohol: Alcohol can irritate the digestive system and cause acid reflux symptoms.

Theobromine, which is present in chocolate, can relax the sphincter muscle at the top of the stomach, allowing stomach acid to reflux into the esophagus.

It is essential to keep in mind that everyone's experience with acid reflux is different, and what works for one person may not work for another. Therefore, it is essential to keep a food and symptom diary and collaborate with your healthcare team to develop a personalized plan for acid reflux management.

In conclusion, the acid reflux diet is an effective way to reduce the frequency and severity of acid reflux symptoms by avoiding or limiting trigger foods and increasing the consumption of digestive-friendly foods. By adhering to this diet and collaborating with your healthcare team, you can achieve equilibrium and enhance your quality of life.

In the following chapter, we will discuss the significance of portion control and meal timing in the acid reflux diet, as well as how to make healthy choices when dining out or on the go.

CHAPTER 4

The Acid Reflux Diet, Including Healthy Fats, Fiber, and Probiotics

In addition to incorporating healthy fats, fiber, and probiotics into your diet, there are a few other methods for controlling acid reflux symptoms. Here are a few starting point suggestions:

Eat smaller, more frequent meals. Large meals can put pressure on the LES, causing acid reflux symptoms. By consuming smaller, more frequent meals throughout the day, you can aid digestion and alleviate symptoms.

Chew your food completely. Taking the time to chew your food thoroughly can facilitate digestion by breaking down food particles into smaller pieces. In addition, thoroughly chewing your food can help stimulate the release of digestive enzymes, thereby enhancing digestion and reducing acid reflux symptoms.

Avoid trigger foods. Certain foods, including fatty foods, fried foods, citrus fruits, tomato-based foods, chocolate, and alcohol, can cause acid reflux symptoms. By identifying your food triggers and avoiding them, you can reduce your symptoms and improve your digestive health overall.

Caffeine and carbonated drinks should be limited. Caffeine and carbonated beverages can induce acid reflux symptoms by exerting pressure on the LES. To reduce symptoms, it is recommended to limit or avoid consumption of these beverages.

Practice stress management techniques. Stress can contribute to acid reflux symptoms by increasing stomach acid production. By engaging in stress management techniques, such as deep breathing, meditation, or yoga, you can reduce symptoms and improve your digestive health overall.

In conclusion, the acid reflux diet is centered on achieving equilibrium. You can reduce symptoms and improve your quality of life by incorporating healthy fats, fiber, and probiotics into your diet, as well as by eating smaller meals, chewing your food thoroughly, and practicing stress management techniques. Managing acid reflux can be simple and efficient with the right approach.

Managing Symptoms with Lifestyle Changes

In addition to dietary adjustments, there are several lifestyle modifications that can be made to alleviate acid reflux symptoms. In this chapter, we will examine some of the most effective methods for managing symptoms and improving digestive health as a whole.

Uphold a Healthy Weight

Maintaining a healthy weight is essential for the management of acid reflux, as excess weight can place pressure on the LES and cause symptoms. You can reduce symptoms and improve overall digestive health by losing weight through a combination of diet and exercise.

Noting that sudden weight loss can trigger symptoms, it is advised to make changes gradually. In addition, if you are considering a weight loss program, you should consult your doctor to ensure that it is safe and effective for you.

Avoid Eating Late at Night

Eating before bedtime can exert pressure on the LES and provoke acid reflux symptoms. It is recommended to avoid eating at least two hours before bedtime to reduce symptoms. If you feel the need for a nighttime snack, choose a low-fat, low-calorie option that will not trigger symptoms.

Raise Your Head While You Sleep

While sleeping, lying flat can put pressure on the LES and cause acid reflux symptoms. To alleviate symptoms, it is recommended to sleep with your head elevated. This can be accomplished by using a pillow or by sleeping on a bed with an adjustable headrest.

Quit Smoking

Smoking can contribute to acid reflux symptoms by relaxing the LES and increasing stomach acid production. To reduce symptoms and improve overall digestive health, quitting smoking is recommended. Your physician can recommend effective cessation methods, such as nicotine replacement therapy and support groups.

Limit Alcohol Consumption

Alcohol can relax the LES and cause acid reflux symptoms. To reduce symptoms, it is recommended to limit or avoid alcohol consumption. If you choose to consume alcohol, choose a low-alcohol beverage and drink plenty of water to stay hydrated.

In conclusion, managing acid reflux symptoms through lifestyle modifications can have a significant impact on enhancing digestive health as a whole. By making changes such as maintaining a healthy weight, avoiding eating before bedtime, sleeping with your head elevated, quitting smoking, and consuming less alcohol, you can reduce symptoms and enhance your quality of life. Controlling acid reflux can be simple and effective if the correct approach is taken.

In addition to the aforementioned lifestyle modifications, there are a number of other strategies for managing acid reflux symptoms.

Reduce Tension

Stress can cause acid reflux symptoms by increasing the production of stomach acid. To reduce symptoms, it is essential to find stress management techniques. This may include physical activity, meditation, or deep breathing. You can also speak with a therapist or counselor to address any emotional issues that may be contributing to your stress.

Keep hydrated

By neutralizing stomach acid, drinking copious amounts of water can reduce acid reflux symptoms. Aim for at least eight glasses of water per day and avoid drinking large quantities of fluid with meals, as this can increase pressure on the LES and cause symptoms.

Avoid Trigger Foods

In addition to making lifestyle adjustments, it is essential to identify and avoid foods that can contribute to acid reflux symptoms. Common dietary triggers include fatty or spicy foods, chocolate, coffee, alcoholic beverages, and carbonated beverages. A food diary can help you determine which foods trigger your symptoms, allowing you to make dietary adjustments accordingly.

Maintain Correct Posture

Inadequate posture can put pressure on the LES and cause acid reflux symptoms. For symptom reduction, it is essential to maintain good posture throughout the day, whether sitting, standing, or sleeping. If necessary, consider using a supportive chair or back brace to improve posture.

Get Regular Exercise

Regular exercise can improve overall digestive health and alleviate acid reflux symptoms. Aim for at least 30 minutes of moderate-intensity physical activity per day, such as brisk walking, swimming, or cycling. Avoid high-impact activities, such as running and jumping, as they can place pressure on the LES and cause symptoms.

In conclusion, there are numerous ways to manage acid reflux symptoms, including modifying your lifestyle, avoiding trigger foods, and engaging in regular exercise. You can gain control of your symptoms and improve your digestive health with the right approach. By making positive changes and adopting a healthy lifestyle, you can enjoy a happier, healthier future and live your best life.

CHAPTER 5

Acid Reflux Complications and Dangers

Acid reflux, also referred to as gastroesophageal reflux disease (GERD), is a common digestive disorder affecting millions of people. Despite the fact that it is typically a mild and manageable condition, if left untreated it can result in a number of serious complications and risks. In this chapter, we will discuss the potential risks and complications of acid reflux, as well as what you can do to prevent or treat them.

Esophagitis

Esophagitis, an inflammation of the esophagus caused by frequent exposure to stomach acid, is one of the most typical complications of acid reflux. Esophagitis can cause heartburn, chest pain, difficulty swallowing, and regurgitation, among other symptoms. Esophagitis can lead to more serious conditions, such as esophageal ulcers and strictures, which can make swallowing difficult and increase the risk of complications, if left untreated.

Barrett's Esophagus

Barrett's esophagus is a condition in which damaged esophageal cells are replaced by abnormal cells. This condition is caused by repeated and prolonged exposure to stomach acid and can increase the risk of esophageal cancer. Barrett's esophagus is characterized by heartburn, chest pain, and difficulty swallowing.

Esophageal Malignancy

Due to long-term exposure to stomach acid, esophageal cancer is a serious and potentially fatal disease that can develop. Esophageal cancer is more prevalent among individuals with Barrett's esophagus and additional risk factors, such as smoking, heavy alcohol consumption, and a family history of the disease. Cancer of the esophagus can manifest as heartburn, chest pain, difficulty swallowing, and weight loss.

Laryngopharyngeal Reflux (LPR)

Laryngopharyngeal reflux (LPR) is a form of acid reflux that affects the throat and voice box. LPR can manifest as hoarseness, coughing, and sore throat. If left untreated, LPR can result in serious complications, including voice changes, breathing difficulties, and aspiration.

Asthma

Asthma symptoms like coughing, wheezing, and shortness of breath can also be triggered by acid reflux. If you have asthma and acid reflux symptoms, it is important to consult a physician, as treatment for acid reflux can help alleviate asthma symptoms.

Prevention and Administration

The best method for preventing and managing acid reflux complications and risks is to treat the underlying condition. This may include weight loss, avoidance of trigger foods, and quitting smoking. In addition, over-the-counter and prescription medications, such as antacids, proton pump inhibitors, and H2 receptor blockers, can assist in alleviating symptoms and preventing complications.

In severe cases, your doctor may recommend surgery to treat acid reflux, such as a laparoscopic Nissen fundoplication. The upper portion of the stomach is wrapped around the lower esophagus to prevent stomach acid from flowing back into the esophagus.

In conclusion, untreated acid reflux can result in a number of serious complications and risks. You can help prevent and manage the complications and risks associated with acid reflux by making lifestyle adjustments, taking prescribed medications, and seeking prompt medical treatment. You can gain control of your symptoms and improve your overall health and well-being with the right approach.

In addition, it is essential to keep track of your symptoms and inform your physician if they change or worsen. Regular examinations and monitoring can aid in early detection and prevention of potential complications.

Maintaining a healthy, low-acid, high-fiber diet is also essential for managing acid reflux. This may entail consuming more fruits, vegetables, and whole grains, as well as avoiding food triggers like spicy, fatty, and acidic foods. Additionally, it is essential to be mindful of portion sizes and to eat slowly, as overeating and eating too quickly can increase the risk of acid reflux.

In addition to dietary modifications, other lifestyle modifications, such as reducing stress and practicing good sleep hygiene, can assist in the management of acid reflux symptoms. Daily exercise, such as a brisk walk or yoga, can also aid digestion and alleviate symptoms.

In some instances, elevated bed frames or acid reflux-specific pillows can be used to prevent acid from flowing back into the esophagus while sleeping. It is essential to discuss these options with your physician in order to determine which one will work best for you.

In the end, achieving equilibrium and managing acid reflux symptoms requires a comprehensive approach that combines medical and lifestyle interventions. By collaborating closely with your physician, making dietary and lifestyle modifications, and adhering to a comprehensive treatment plan, you can effectively manage your symptoms and reduce your risk of complications.

CHAPTER 6

Everyday Acid Reflux Management

Living with acid reflux can be difficult, but there are several strategies that can help you manage the symptoms and effectively live with the condition. In this chapter, we will discuss some of these techniques and offer advice on how to live a full and active life despite acid reflux.

Keeping a daily record of your symptoms can be useful for identifying triggers and patterns, as well as for discussing your progress with your doctor. Make a record of the foods you eat, the times you experience symptoms, and any other factors that appear to affect your acid reflux.

Certain foods and activities can trigger acid reflux symptoms, so it is important to identify your triggers and avoid them whenever possible. Common allergen triggers include fatty or spicy foods, chocolate, caffeine, alcoholic beverages, and tobacco.

Adopt Healthy Eating Habits: Eating smaller, more frequent meals and chewing food thoroughly can help reduce symptoms. Consider elevating the head of your bed to prevent acid from flowing back into your esophagus while you are sleeping.

Stress can be a trigger for acid reflux; therefore, finding ways to manage stress, such as through exercise, meditation, or therapy, can be beneficial for alleviating symptoms.

Regular physical activity can improve digestion and reduce symptoms, but it is important to avoid abdominal-pressing exercises, such as heavy lifting and running.

Seek Support: Speaking with friends, family, or a support group can offer emotional support and reduce feelings of isolation. Joining a support group can also provide valuable information and guidance from those who have faced comparable obstacles.

It is essential to have an open and honest conversation with your doctor about your symptoms, treatment options, and any concerns you may have. In addition to providing guidance and support, your physician can adjust your treatment plan as necessary.

By implementing the aforementioned strategies, you can effectively manage your acid reflux symptoms and continue to live a full and active life.

Remember that everyone's experience with acid reflux is different, so it is essential to work closely with your doctor to determine the strategies that will be most effective for you. You can effectively manage your acid reflux and live a healthy, happy life with the help of proper treatment and a comprehensive strategy.

In addition, it is essential to educate yourself about acid reflux and stay abreast of the most recent treatment developments. This can empower you to take an active role in managing your condition and assist you in making informed decisions regarding your care.

In addition, it is essential to prioritize self-care and develop healthy self-management practices, such as staying hydrated, obtaining sufficient rest, and avoiding late-night snacking. By taking care of your health and wellbeing as a whole, you can alleviate your symptoms and reduce your risk of complications.

In some instances, over-the-counter antacids or prescription medications may be required to manage symptoms of acid reflux. It is essential to follow your doctor's instructions and use medications as prescribed. If you experience side effects or a worsening of your symptoms, it is essential to discuss these with your doctor as soon as possible.

Even during difficult times, it is important to maintain a positive outlook and remain optimistic. Living with acid reflux can be difficult, but there are numerous strategies and treatments that can help you manage your symptoms and live a healthy, fulfilling life. You can overcome the difficulties of acid reflux and enjoy a higher quality of life with the right support and a comprehensive approach.

CONCLUSION

The Challenges of Living with Acid Reflux

It can be challenging to live with acid reflux, but it is possible to effectively manage symptoms and lead a healthy and fulfilling life with the right approach. This book discusses the causes, symptoms, and treatments for acid reflux, as well as daily coping strategies.

The key to effective management of acid reflux is collaborating closely with your doctor to develop an individualized, comprehensive treatment plan. This may involve dietary and physical activity modifications, as well as, if necessary, medication.

Additionally, it is essential to educate yourself about the condition, remain current on the latest developments, and seek support when necessary. Having a supportive network, whether through a support group, friends, family, or therapy, can provide emotional support and help you feel less isolated.

In addition, it is crucial to prioritize self-care and engage in regular self-management practices, such as staying hydrated, obtaining sufficient rest, and avoiding late-night snacking. By taking care of your health and wellbeing as a whole, you can alleviate your symptoms and reduce your risk of complications.

Despite the difficulty of living with acid reflux, it is essential to maintain a positive outlook and remain optimistic, even during difficult times. You can overcome the difficulties of acid reflux and enjoy a higher quality of life with the right support and a comprehensive approach.

Remember that everyone's experience with acid reflux is different, and it is essential to work closely with your doctor to determine which strategies will work best for you. You can effectively manage your acid reflux and lead a healthy, happy life with the help of proper treatment and a comprehensive strategy.

www.ingramcontent.com/pod-product-compliance
Lightning Source LLC
Chambersburg PA
CBHW061616250726
48653CB00016B/3081